Quick and Easy Keto Vegetarian Recipes

Easy and Delicious Low-Carb, Plant-Based Recipes to Lose Weight and Feel Great

Dr. William Coleman

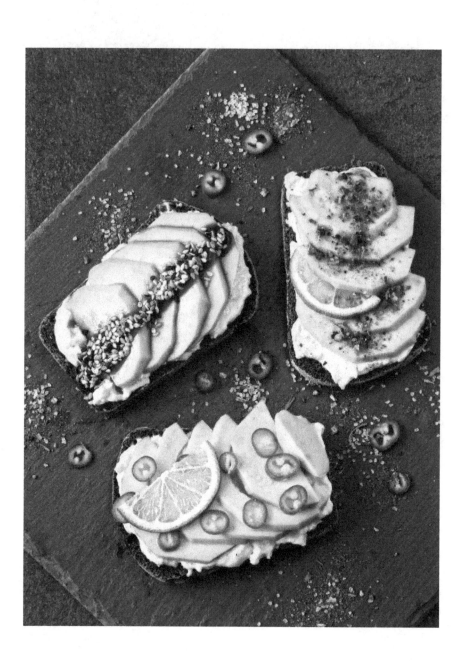

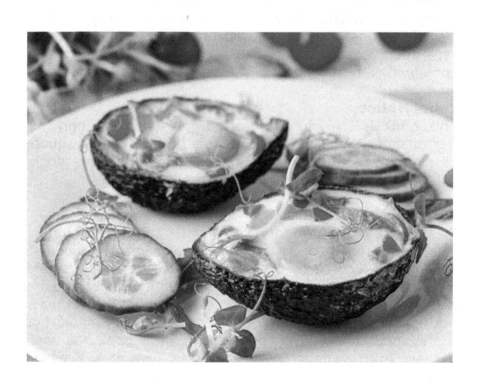

TABLE OF CONTENTS

INTRODUCTION

Essentially, a ketogenic diet is a diet that drastically restricts your carb intake and fat intake; this pushes your body to go into a state of ketosis.

Your body uses glucose from carbs to fuel metabolic pathways—meaning various bodily functions like digestion, breathing—essentially anything that needs energy. Glucose is therefore the primary pathway when it comes to sourcing the body's energy.

But the body has also another pathway, it can make use of fats to fuel the various bodily processes. And this is what is called ketosis. The body can only enter ketosis when there is no glucose available, thus the reason why eating a low-carb diet is essential in the keto diet.

Since no glucose is available, the body is pushed to use fats—it can either come from the food you consume or from your body's fat reserves—the adipose tissue or from the flabby parts of your body. This is how the keto diet helps you lose weight, by burning up all those stored fats that you have and using it to fuel bodily processes.

Ketosis is a very natural process, the body will soon adapt to this state and therefore you will be able to lose weight in no time but you will also become healthier and your physical and mental performances will improve. Your blood sugar levels will improve and you won't be predisposed to diabetes. Also, epilepsy and heart disease can be easily be prevented if you are on a ketogenic diet. Your cholesterol will improve and you will feel amazing in no time. How does that sound?

That said, if for whatever reason you are a vegetarian, following a ketogenic diet can be extremely difficult. A vegetarian diet is largely free of animal products, which means that food tends to be usually high in carbohydrates. Still, with careful planning, it is possible.

This Cookbook will provide you with various easy and delicious dishes to help you stick to your ketogenic diet plan while being a vegetarian.

Enjoy!

Almond English Muffins

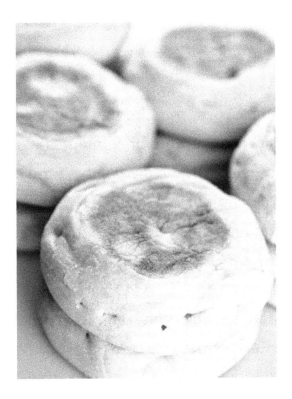

Preparation Time: 10 minutes

Cooking Time: 10 minutes

Serving: 4

Ingredients:

- 2 tbsp flax seed powder + 6 tbsp water
- 2 tbsp almond flour

- ½ tsp baking powder
- 1 pinch salt
- 3 tbsp butter

Directions:

1. In a small bowl, mix the flax seed with water and allow thickening for 5 minutes.
2. In another bowl, evenly combine the almond flour, baking powder, and salt. Then, pour in the flax egg and whisk again. Let the batter sit for 5 minutes to set.
3. Melt the butter in a frying pan over medium heat and add the mixture in four dollops with 1-inch intervals between each dollop. Fry until golden brown on one side, flip with a spatula and fry further until golden brown.
4. Plate the muffins and serve warm.

Nutrition:

Calories: 263, Total Fat: 26.4g, Saturated Fat:9.5 g, Total Carbs: 4 g, Dietary Fiber: 4g, Sugar:3 g, Protein:4 g, Sodium: 826mg

Blueberry Soufflé

Preparation Time: 15 minutes

Cooking Time: 20 minutes

Serving: 4

Ingredients:

For the blueberry sauce:

- 1 cup frozen blueberries
- 2 tsp erythritol
- 1 tbsp water

For the omelet:

- 4 egg yolks, room temperature
- 3 tbsp erythritol, divided
- 3 egg whites, room temperature
- 1 tsp olive oil
- ½ lemon, zested to garnish

Directions:

For the blueberry sauce:

1. Pour the blueberries, erythritol and water in a small saucepan over medium heat.

2. Cook with occasional stirring until the berries soften and become syrupy, 8 to 10 minutes. Stir in the vanilla, turn the heat off, and set aside to cool slightly.

For the omelet:

3. Preheat the oven to 350 ⁰F.
4. In a large bowl, beat the egg yolks and 1 tablespoon of erythritol with an electric whisk until thick and pale.
5. In another bowl, whisk the egg whites at low speed with clean beaters until foamy. Increase the speed, add the remaining erythritol, 1 tablespoon at a time, and whisk until soft peak forms, 3 to 4 minutes.
6. Gently and gradually, fold the egg white mixture into the egg yolk mix.
7. Heat the olive oil in a safe oven non-stick frying pan over low heat. Swirl the pan to spread the oil and pour in the egg mixture; swirl to spread too.
8. Cook for 3 minutes and then, transfer to the oven; bake for 2 to 3 minutes or until golden, puffed, and set.

9. Plate the omelet and spoon the blueberry sauce onto the egg.
10. Use the spoon to spread around. Garnish with lemon zest.
11. Serve immediately with tea or coffee.

Nutrition:

Calories:478, Total Fat: 46.8g, Saturated Fat:27.3 g, Total Carbs: 8 g, Dietary Fiber: 4g, Sugar: 1g, Protein: 11g, Sodium: 257mg

Spinach and Cucumber Salad

Preparation time: 5 minutes

Cooking time: 0 minutes

Servings: 4

Ingredients:

- 1 pound cucumber, sliced
- 2 cups baby spinach
- 1 tablespoon chili powder
- 2 tablespoons olive oil
- ¼ cup cilantro, chopped
- 2 tablespoons lemon juice
- Salt and black pepper to the taste

Directions:

1. In a large salad bowl, combine the cucumber with the spinach and the other ingredients, toss and serve for lunch.

Nutrition:

calories 140, fat 4, fiber 2, carbs 4, protein 5

Greens and Olives Pan

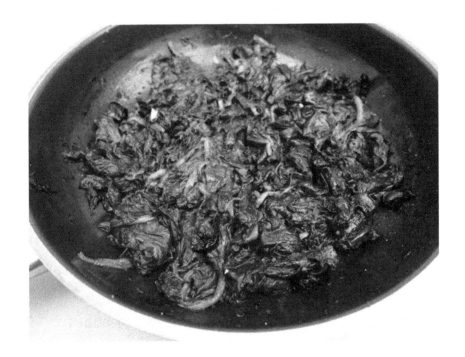

Preparation time: 10 minutes

Cooking time: 15 minutes

Servings: 4

Ingredients:

- 4 spring onions, chopped
- 2 tablespoons olive oil
- ½ cup green olives, pitted and halved

- ¼ cup pine nuts, toasted
- 1 tablespoon balsamic vinegar
- 2 cups baby spinach
- 1 cup baby arugula
- 1 cup asparagus, trimmed, blanched and halved
- Salt and black pepper to the taste

Directions:

1. Heat up a pan with the oil over medium high heat, add the spring onions and the asparagus and sauté for 5 minutes.
2. Add the olives, spinach and the other ingredients, toss, cook over medium heat for 10 minutes, divide between plates and serve for lunch.

Nutrition:

calories 136, fat 13.1, fiber 1.9, carbs 4.4, protein 2.8

Broccoli, Chard and Kale Mix

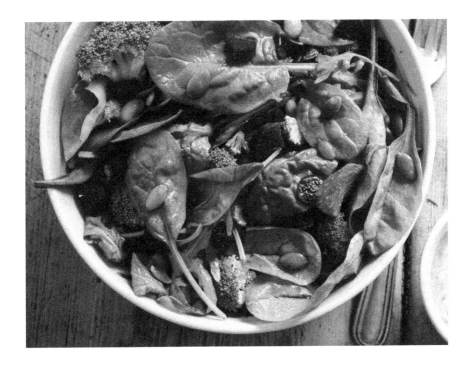

Preparation time: 10 minutes

Cooking time: 20 minutes

Servings: 4

Ingredients:

- ½ cup kale, torn
- 2 cups red chard, torn
- 2 cups broccoli florets

- 4 garlic cloves, minced
- 2 tablespoons olive oil
- 1 tablespoon balsamic vinegar
- 1 tablespoon lemon juice
- ½ cup almonds, sliced
- 1 tablespoon chives, chopped

Directions:

1. In a roasting pan, combine the kale with the chard, broccoli and the other ingredients, toss and bake at 400 degrees F for 20 minutes.
2. Divide everything between plates and serve right away.

Nutrition:

calories 90, fat 1, fiber 3, carbs 7, protein 2

Mashed Cauliflower

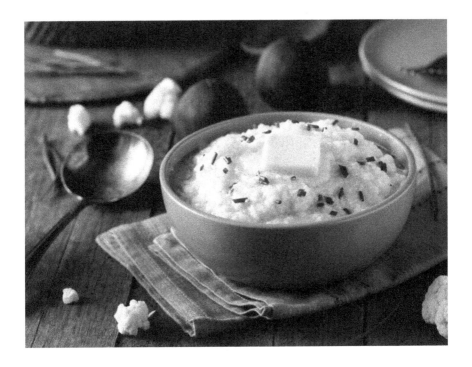

Preparation Time: 10 minutes

Cooking Time: 15 minutes

Servings: 6

Ingredients:

- 2 tablespoons milk
- 4 tablespoons butter
- 2 cauliflower heads, cut into florets

- ½ teaspoon onion powder
- ½ teaspoon garlic powder
- ½ teaspoon sea salt
- ½ teaspoon pepper

Directions:

1. Add your cauliflower to a saucepan filled with enough water to cover the cauliflower. Cook cauliflower over medium heat for 15 minutes. Drain your cauliflower florets and place it in a mixing bowl. Add remaining ingredients to the bowl. Using a blender blend until smooth. Serve and enjoy!

Nutritional Values (Per Serving):

Calories: 120 Fat: 8 g Cholesterol: 21 mg Sugar: 5 g Carbohydrates: 10.9 g Protein: 4.1 g

Roasted Green Beans

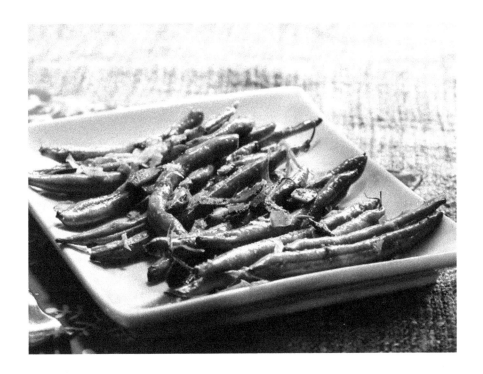

Preparation Time: 15 minutes

Cooking Time: 30 minutes

Servings: 4

Ingredients:

- 1 lb. green beans, frozen
- 2 tablespoons extra-virgin olive oil

- ½ teaspoon onion powder
- ½ teaspoon garlic powder
- ½ teaspoon sea salt
- ½ teaspoon pepper

Directions:

1. Preheat your oven to 425°Fahrenheit. Spray a cooking tray with cooking spray. In a bowl add all your ingredients and mix well. Spread the green beans on the prepared baking tray and bake for 30 minutes. Serve and enjoy!

Nutritional Values (Per Serving):

Calories: 98 Sugar: 1.8 g Carbohydrates: 8.8 g Fat: 7.2 g Cholesterol: 0 mg Protein: 2.2 g

Gluten Free Asparagus Quiche

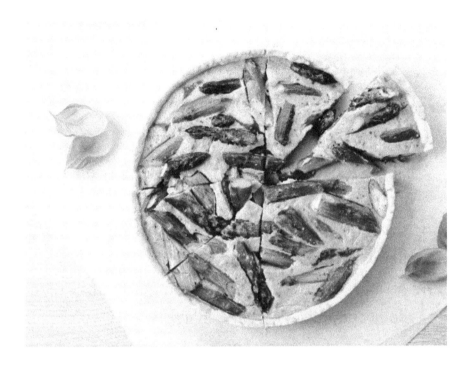

Preparation Time: 1 hour 10 minutes

Servings: 6

Ingredients:

- 5 eggs, beaten
- 1 cup Swiss cheese, shredded
- 1/4 tsp thyme
- 1/4 tsp white pepper

- 1 cup almond milk
- 15 asparagus spears, cut woody ends and cut asparagus in half
- 1/4 tsp salt

Directions:

1. Preheat the oven to 350 F.
2. Spray a quiche dish with cooking spray and set aside.
3. In a bowl, beat together eggs, thyme, white pepper, almond milk, and salt.
4. Arrange asparagus in prepared quiche dish then pour egg mixture over asparagus.
5. Sprinkle shredded cheese all over asparagus and egg mixture.
6. Place in preheated oven and bake for 60 minutes.
7. Cut quiche into slices and serve.

Nutritional Value (Amount per Serving):

Calories 225 Fat 18 g Carbohydrates 5 g Sugar 3 g Protein 11 g Cholesterol 153 mg

Braised Seitan with Kelp Noodles

Preparation Time: 10 minutes

Cooking Time: 2 hours 2 minutes

Serving: 4

Ingredients:

- 1 tbsp olive oil
- 2 pieces star anise
- 1 cinnamon stick
- 1 garlic clove, minced
- 1-inch ginger, grated
- 1 ½ lb seitan, cut into strips
- 3 tbsp tamarind sauce
- 2 tbsp swerve sugar
- ¼ cup red wine
- ¼ cup water
- 4 cups vegetable broth
- 2 (23.9oz) kelp noodles, thoroughly rinsed
- For topping:
- 1 cup steamed napa cabbage
- Scallions, thinly sliced

Directions:

1. Heat the olive oil in a medium pot over medium

heat and stir-fry the star anise, cinnamon, garlic, and ginger until fragrant, 5 minutes.

2. Mix in the seitan, season with salt, black pepper, and sear on both sides, 10 minutes.

3. In a small bowl, combine the tamarind sauce, swerve sugar, red wine, and water. Pour the mixture into the pot, close the lid, and bring to a boil. Reduce the heat and simmer for 30 to 45 minutes or until the seitan is tender.

4. Strain the pot's content through a colander into a bowl and pour the braising liquid back into the pot. Discard the cinnamon, star anise and set the seitan aside.

5. Add the vegetable broth to the pot and simmer until hot, 10 minutes.

6. Put the kelp noodles into the broth and cook until softened and separated, 5 to 7 minutes.

7. Spoon the noodles with some broth into serving bowls, top with the seitan strips, and then the cabbage and scallions.

Nutrition:

Calories: 311, Total Fat: 18g, Saturated Fat: 6.3g, Total Carbs: 3 g, Dietary Fiber:0 g, Sugar:2 g, Protein:34 g, Sodium:136 mg

Seitan Tex-Mex Casserole

Preparation Time: 5 minutes

Cooking Time: 35 minutes

Serving: 4

Ingredients:

- 2 tbsp butter
- 1 ½ lb seitan
- 3 tbsp Tex-Mex seasoning
- 2 tbsp chopped jalapeño peppers
- ½ cup crushed tomatoes
- Salt and black pepper to taste
- ½ cup shredded provolone cheese
- 1 tbsp chopped fresh green onion to garnish
- 1 cup sour cream for serving

Directions:

1. Preheat the oven and grease a baking dish with cooking spray. Set aside.
2. Melt the butter in a medium skillet over medium heat and cook the seitan until brown, 10 minutes.

3. Stir in the Tex-Mex seasoning, jalapeño peppers, and tomatoes; simmer for 5 minutes and adjust the taste with salt and black pepper.
4. Transfer and level the mixture in the baking dish. Top with the provolone cheese and bake in the upper rack of the oven for 15 to 20 minutes or until the cheese melts and is golden brown.
5. Remove the dish and garnish with the green onion.
6. Serve the casserole with sour cream.

Nutrition:

Calories: 464, Total Fat:37.8 g, Saturated Fat:7.4 g, Total Carbs: 12 g, Dietary Fiber: 2g, Sugar: 3g, Protein:24 g, Sodium: 147mg

Tempeh Coconut Curry Bake

Preparation Time: 7 minutes

Cooking Time: 23 minutes

Serving: 4

Ingredients:

- 1 oz. plant butter, for greasing
- 2 ½ cups chopped tempeh
- Salt and black pepper
- 4 tbsp plant butter
- 2 tbsp red curry paste
- 1 ½ cup coconut cream
- ½ cup fresh parsley, chopped
- 15 oz. cauliflower, cut into florets

Directions:

1. Preheat the oven to 400 F and grease a baking dish with 1 ounce of butter.
2. Arrange the tempeh in the baking dish, sprinkle with salt and black pepper, and top each tempeh with a slice of the remaining butter.

3. In a bowl, mix the red curry paste with the coconut cream and parsley. Pour the mixture over the tempeh.
4. Bake in the oven for 20 minutes or until the tempeh is cooked.
5. While baking, season the cauliflower with salt, place in a microwave-safe bowl, and sprinkle with some water. Steam in the microwave for 3 minutes or until the cauliflower is soft and tender within.
6. Remove the curry bake and serve with the caulis.

Nutrition:

Calories:417, Total Fat:38.8g, Saturated Fat:22.4g, Total Carbs: 11g, Dietary Fiber:2g, Sugar: 3g, Protein: 11g, Sodium: 194mg

Cauliflower Salad

Preparation time: 10 minutes

Cooking time: 0 minutes

Servings: 4

Ingredients:

- 1 pound cauliflower florets, blanched
- 1 avocado, peeled, pitted and cubed
- 1 cup kalamata olives, pitted and halved
- Salt and black pepper to the taste
- 1 cup spring onions, chopped
- 1 tablespoon lime juice
- 1 tablespoon chives, chopped

Directions:

1. In a bowl, combine the cauliflower florets with the avocado and the other ingredients, toss and serve as a side salad.

Nutrition:

calories 211, fat 20, fiber 2, carbs 3, protein 4

Orange Carrots

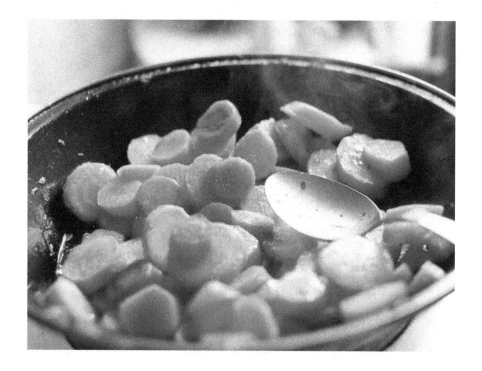

Preparation time: 5 minutes

Cooking time: 25 minutes

Servings: 4

Ingredients:

- 1 pound carrots, peeled and roughly sliced
- 1 yellow onion, chopped
- 1 tablespoon olive oil

- Zest of 1 orange, grated
- Juice of 1 orange
- 1 orange, peeled and cut into segments
- 1 tablespoon rosemary, chopped
- A pinch of salt and black pepper

Directions:

1. Heat up a pan with the oil over medium-high heat, add the onion and sauté for 5 minutes.
2. Add the carrots, the orange zest and the other ingredients, toss, cook over medium heat for 20 minutes more, divide between plates and serve.

Nutrition:

calories 140, fat 3.9, fiber 5, carbs 26.1, protein 2.1

Quinoa and Peas

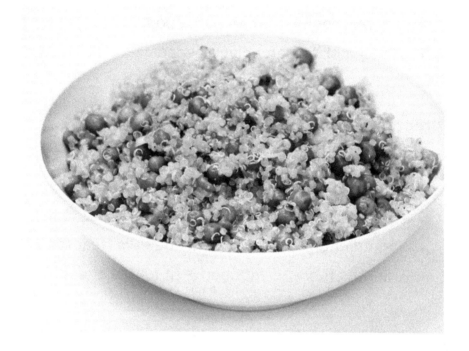

Preparation time: 10 minutes

Cooking time: 30 minutes

Servings: 4

Ingredients:

- 1 yellow onion, chopped
- 1 tomato, cubed
- 1 cup quinoa

- 3 cups vegetable stock
- 1 tablespoon olive oil
- 1 cup peas
- 1 tablespoon cilantro, chopped
- A pinch of salt and black pepper

Directions:

1. Heat up a pot with the oil over medium heat, add the onion, stir and sauté for 5 minutes.
2. Add the quinoa, the stock and the other ingredients, toss, bring to a simmer and cook over medium heat for 25 minutes.
3. Divide everything between plates and serve as a side dish.

Nutrition:

calories 202, fat 3, fiber 3, carbs 11, protein 6

Basil Green Beans

Preparation time: 10 minutes

Cooking time: 20 minutes

Servings: 4

Ingredients:

- 1 yellow onion, chopped
- 1 pound green beans, trimmed and halved
- 1 tablespoon avocado oil
- 2 teaspoons basil, dried
- A pinch of salt and black pepper
- 1 tablespoon tomato sauce

Directions:

1. Heat up a pan with the oil over medium-high heat, add the onion and sauté for 5 minutes.
2. Add the green beans and the other ingredients, toss, cook for 15 minutes more.
3. Divide everything between plates and serve as a side dish.

Nutrition:

calories 221, fat 5, fiber 8, carbs 10, protein 8

Beet and Cabbage

Preparation time: 10 minutes

Cooking time: 20 minutes

Servings: 4

Ingredients:

- 1 green cabbage head, shredded
- 1 yellow onion, chopped
- 1 beet, peeled and cubed
- ½ cup chicken stock
- 2 tablespoons olive oil
- A pinch of salt and black pepper
- 2 tablespoons chives, chopped

Directions:

1. Heat up a pan with the oil over medium heat, add the onion and sauté for 5 minutes.
2. Add the cabbage and the other ingredients, toss, cook over medium heat for 15 minutes more, divide between plates and serve.

Nutrition:

calories 128, fat 7.3, fiber 5.6, carbs 15.6, protein 3.1

Coriander Black Beans

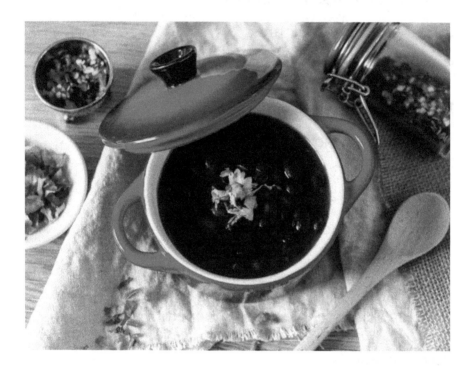

Preparation time: 10 minutes

Cooking time: 20 minutes

Servings: 4

Ingredients:

- 1 tablespoon olive oil
- 2 cups canned black beans, drained and rinsed
- 1 green bell pepper, chopped

- 1 yellow onion, chopped
- 4 garlic cloves, minced
- 1 teaspoon cumin, ground
- ½ cup chicken stock
- 1 tablespoon coriander, chopped
- A pinch of salt and black pepper

Directions:

1. Heat up a pan with the oil over medium heat, add the onion and the garlic and sauté for 5 minutes.
2. Add the black beans and the other ingredients, toss, cook over medium heat for 15 minutes more, divide between plates and serve.

Nutrition:

calories 221, fat 5, fiber 4, carbs 9, protein 11

Garlic Asparagus and Tomatoes

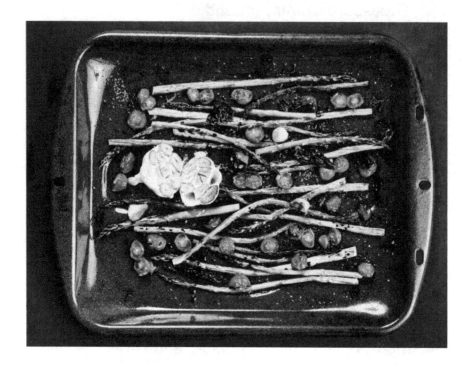

Preparation time: 10 minutes

Cooking time: 20 minutes

Servings: 4

Ingredients:

- 1 pound asparagus, trimmed and halved
- ½ pound cherry tomatoes, halved
- 2 tablespoons olive oil

- 1 teaspoon turmeric powder
- 2 tablespoons shallot, chopped
- A pinch of salt and black pepper
- 1 tablespoon chives, chopped

Directions:

1. Spread the asparagus on a baking sheet lined with parchment paper, add the tomatoes and the other ingredients, toss, cook in the oven at 375 degrees F for 20 minutes.
2. Divide everything between plates and serve as a side dish.

Nutrition:

calories 132, fat 1, fiber 2, carbs 4, protein 4

Sage Quinoa

Preparation time: 10 minutes

Cooking time: 30 minutes

Servings: 4

Ingredients:

- 1 tablespoon olive oil
- 1 yellow onion, chopped
- 1 cup quinoa
- 2 cups chicken stock
- 1 tablespoon sage, chopped
- 2 garlic cloves, minced
- A pinch of salt and black pepper
- 1 tablespoon chives, chopped

Directions:

1. Heat up a pan with the oil over medium-high heat, add the onion and the garlic and sauté for 5 minutes.
2. Add the quinoa and the other ingredients, toss, cook over medium heat for 25 minutes more, divide between plates and serve.

Nutrition:

calories 182, fat 1, fiber 1, carbs 11, protein 8

Glazed Curried Carrots

Preparation time: 5 minutes

cooking time: 15 minutes

servings: 6

Ingredients

- 1 pound carrots, peeled and thinly sliced
- 2 tablespoons olive oil
- 2 tablespoons curry powder
- 2 tablespoons pure maple syrup
- juice of ½ lemon
- sea salt
- freshly ground black pepper

Directions

1. Place the carrots in a large pot and cover with water. Cook on medium-high heat until tender, about 10 minutes. Drain the carrots and return them to the pan over medium-low heat.
2. Stir in the olive oil, curry powder, maple syrup, and lemon juice. Cook, stirring constantly, until the liquid reduces, about 5 minutes. Season with salt and pepper and serve immediately.

Watercress Soup

Preparation time: 10 minutes

Cooking time: 20 minutes

Servings: 4

Ingredients:

- 8 ounces watercress
- 1 tablespoon lemon juice
- A pinch of nutmeg, ground
- 4 ounces coconut milk
- A pinch of sea salt
- Black pepper to taste
- 14 ounces veggie stock
- 1 celery stick, chopped
- 1 onion, chopped
- 1 tablespoon olive oil
- 12 ounces sweet potatoes, peeled and chopped

Directions:

1. Heat up a large saucepan with the oil over medium heat, add onion and celery, stir and cook for 5 minutes.

2. Add sweet potato pieces and stock, stir, bring to a simmer, cover and cook on a low heat for 10 minutes.
3. Add watercress, stir, cover saucepan again and cook for 5 minutes.
4. Blend this with an immersion blender, add a pinch of nutmeg, lemon juice, salt, pepper and coconut milk, bring to a simmer again, divide into bowls and serve.
5. Enjoy!

Nutritional value/serving:

calories 224, fat 11,8, fiber 5,7, carbs 29,6, protein 4

Celery Stew

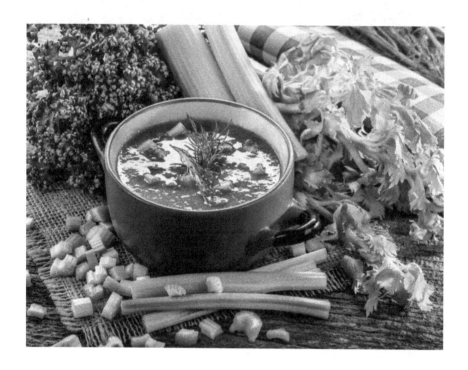

Preparation time: 10 minutes

Cooking time: 30 minutes

Servings: 6

Ingredients:

- 1 celery bunch, chopped
- 1 onion, peeled and chopped
- 1 bunch green onion, peeled and chopped

- 4 garlic cloves, peeled and minced
- Salt and ground black pepper, to taste
- 1 fresh parsley bunch, chopped
- 2 fresh mint bunches, chopped
- 3 dried Persian lemons, pricked with a fork
- 2 cups water
- 2 teaspoons chicken bouillon
- 4 tablespoons olive oil

Directions:

1. Heat up a pot with the oil over medium-high heat, add the onion, green onions, and garlic, stir, and cook for 6 minutes.
2. Add the celery, Persian lemons, chicken bouillon, salt, pepper, and water, stir, cover pot, and simmer on medium heat for 20 minutes.
3. Add the parsley and mint, stir, and cook for 10 minutes.
4. Divide into bowls and serve.

Nutrition:

Calories - 170, Fat - 7, Fiber - 4, Carbs - 6, Protein - 10

Asparagus and Browned Butter

Preparation time: 10 minutes

Cooking time: 15 minutes

Servings: 4

Ingredients:

- 5 ounces butter
- 1 tablespoon avocado oil
- 1½ pounds asparagus, trimmed
- 1½ tablespoons lemon juice
- A pinch of cayenne pepper
- 8 tablespoons sour cream
- Salt and ground black pepper, to taste
- 3 ounces Parmesan cheese, grated
- 4 eggs

Directions:

1. Heat up a pan with 2 ounces butter over medium-high heat, add the eggs, some salt and pepper, stir, and scramble them.
2. Transfer the eggs to a blender, add the Parmesan cheese, sour cream, salt, pepper, and

cayenne pepper, and blend everything well.

3. Heat up a pan with the oil over medium-high heat, add the asparagus, salt, and pepper, roast for a few minutes, transfer to a plate, and set aside.

4. Heat up the pan again with the rest of the butter over medium-high heat, stir until brown, take off the heat, add the lemon juice, and stir well.

5. Heat up the butter again, return the asparagus to the pan, toss to coat, heat up well, and divide on plates.

6. Add the blended eggs on top and serve.

Nutrition:

Calories - 160, Fat - 7, Fiber - 2, Carbs - 6, Protein - 10

Alfalfa Sprouts Salad

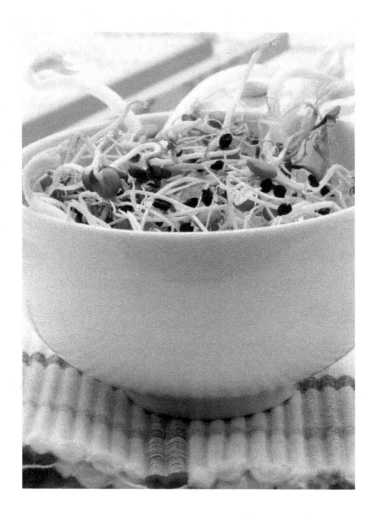

Preparation time: 10 minutes

Cooking time: 0 minutes

Servings: 4

Ingredients:

- 1 green apple, cored, and julienned
- 1½ teaspoons dark sesame oil
- 4 cups alfalfa sprouts
- Salt and ground black pepper, to taste
- 1½ teaspoons grape seed oil
- ¼ cup coconut milk yogurt
- 4 nasturtium leaves

Directions:

1. In a salad bowl, mix the sprouts with apple and nasturtium.
2. Add the salt, pepper, sesame oil, grape seed oil, and coconut yogurt, toss to coat, and divide on plates, and serve.

Nutrition:

Calories - 100, Fat - 3, Fiber - 1, Carbs - 2, Protein - 6

Eggplant Soup

Preparation time: 10 minutes

Cooking time: 50 minutes

Servings: 4

Ingredients:

- 4 tomatoes
- 1 teaspoon garlic, minced
- ¼ onion, peeled and chopped
- Salt and ground black pepper, to taste
- 2 cups chicken stock
- 1 bay leaf
- ½ cup heavy cream
- 2 tablespoons fresh basil, chopped
- 4 tablespoons Parmesan cheese, grated
- 1 tablespoon olive oil
- 1 eggplant, chopped

Directions:

1. Spread the eggplant pieces on a baking sheet, mix with oil, onion, garlic, salt, and pepper, place in an oven at 400ºF, and bake for 15

minutes.

2. Put water in a pot, bring to a boil over medium heat, add the tomatoes, steam them for 1 minute, peel them, and chop.

3. Take the eggplant mixture out of the oven, and transfer to a pot.

4. Add the tomatoes, stock, bay leaf, salt, and pepper, stir, bring to a boil, and simmer for 30 minutes.

5. Add the heavy cream, basil, and Parmesan cheese, stir, ladle into soup bowls, and serve.

Nutrition:

Calories - 180, Fat - 2, Fiber - 3, Carbs - 5, Protein - 10

Roasted Bell Peppers Soup

Preparation time: 10 minutes

Cooking time: 15 minutes

Servings: 6

Ingredients:

- 12 ounces roasted bell peppers, seeded and chopped
- 2 tablespoons olive oil
- 2 garlic cloves, peeled and minced
- 29 ounces canned chicken stock
- Salt and ground black pepper, to taste
- 7 ounces water
- ⅔ cup heavy cream
- 1 onion, peeled and chopped
- ¼ cup Parmesan cheese, grated
- 2 celery stalks, chopped

Directions:

1. Heat up a pot with the oil over medium heat, add the onion, garlic, celery, and some salt, and pepper, stir, and cook for 8 minutes.

2. Add the bell peppers, water, and stock, stir, bring to a boil, cover, reduce the heat, and simmer for 5 minutes.
3. Use an immersion blender to puree the soup, then add more salt, pepper, and cream, stir, bring to a boil, and take off the heat.
4. Ladle into bowls, sprinkle Parmesan cheese, and serve.

Nutrition:

Calories - 176, Fat - 13, Fiber - 1, Carbs - 4, Protein - 6

Crunchy Cauliflower Bites

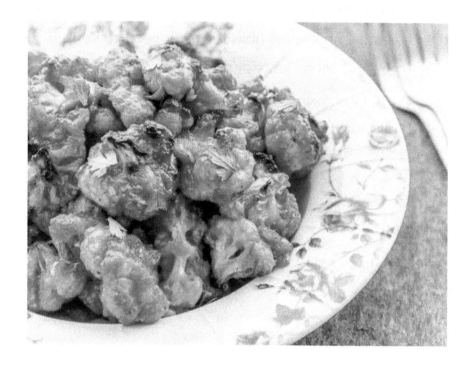

Preparation Time: 10 minutes

Cooking Time: 20 minutes

Servings: 8

Ingredients:

- 2 eggs, organic, beaten
- 1 tablespoon Parmesan cheese, grated
- ½ head cauliflower, cut into florets

- 1 cup breadcrumbs
- Pepper and salt to taste

Directions:

1. Preheat your oven to 395°Fahrenheit. Spray baking dish with cooking spray and set aside. In a shallow dish combine the cheese, breadcrumbs, pepper, and salt. Dip the cauliflower florets in beaten egg then roll in breadcrumb mixture. Place coated cauliflower florets onto prepared baking dish. Bake in preheated oven for 20 minutes. Serve hot and enjoy!

Nutrition:

Calories: 81 Sugar: 1.3 g Fat: 2.4 g Carbohydrates: 10.7 g Cholesterol: 42 mg Protein: 4.3 g

Curry with Bok Choy

Preparation Time: 15 minutes

Cooking Time: 15 minutes

Servings: 3

Ingredients:

- 2 tablespoons extra virgin coconut oil or olive oil
- 1 small onion, peeled, finely diced
- 2 cloves garlic, peeled, finely chopped
- 1 tablespoon curry powder
- 1 tablespoon fresh grated ginger
- ½ teaspoon ground turmeric
- ½ teaspoon ground fenugreek
- 2 bok choy, washed, feet removed, roughly chopped (14 oz.)
- 14 oz. unsweetened coconut milk
- ½ cup vegetable stock

For serving:

- Lemon juice
- Fresh coriander
- Chili flake

Directions:

1. Place a large skillet over medium heat and add oil. Once the oil is heated, add onions and garlic and cook 1-2 minutes or until golden brown, taking care not to burn them.
2. Add curry powder, grated ginger, turmeric and fenugreek. Stir fry 30 seconds to1 minute until fragrant.
3. Stir in bok choy then cover, turn the heat down to medium-low, and cook 3-4 minutes.
4. Increase the heat to medium-high, uncover and cook 3 - 4 minutes to evaporate the vegetable juice slightly.
5. Pour in coconut milk and vegetable stock; cook an additional 10 minutes until a thick liquid reduces.
6. Place curry in a serving bowl. Drizzle with lemon juice. Sprinkle with freshly chopped coriander and chili flakes.

Nutrition:

Calories: 200, Total Fats: 15.3g, Carbohydrates: 13.4g, Fiber: 4.8g, Protein: 4.7g, Sugar: 5.2

Almond Soup With Cardamom

Preparation time: 5 minutes

cooking time: 35 minutes total: 40minutes

servings: 4

Ingredients

- 1 tablespoon olive oil
- 1 medium onion, chopped
- 1 medium russet potato, chopped
- 1 medium red bell pepper, chopped
- 4 cups vegetable broth, homemade (see Light Vegetable Brothor store-bought, or water
- 1/2 teaspoon ground cardamom
- Salt and freshly ground black pepper
- 1/2 cup almond butter
- 1/4 cup sliced toasted almonds, for garnish

Directions

1. In a large soup pot, heat the oil over medium heat. Add the onion, potato, and bell pepper. Cover and cook until softened, about 5 minutes.
2. Add the broth, cardamom, and salt and pepper

to taste. Bring to a boil, then reduce heat to low and simmer, uncovered, until the vegetables are tender, about 30 minutes.

3. Add the almond butter and puree in the pot with an immersion blender or in a blender or food processor, in batches if necessary, and return to the pot.

4. Reheat over medium heat until hot. Taste, adjusting seasonings if necessary, and add more broth or some soy milk if needed for desired consistency.

5. Ladle the soup into bowls, sprinkle with toasted sliced almonds, and serve.

Sweet Potato And Peanut Soup With Baby Spinach

Preparation Time: 5 Minutes

Cooking Time: 40 Minutes

Servings:4

Ingredients

- 1 tablespoon olive oil
- 1 medium onion, chopped
- 11/2 pounds sweet potatoes, peeled and cut into 1/2-inch dice
- 6 cups vegetable broth, homemade (see Light Vegetable Broth) or store-bought, or water
- 1/3 cup creamy peanut butter
- 1/4 teaspoon ground cayenne
- 1/8 teaspoon ground nutmeg
- Salt and freshly ground black pepper
- 4 cups fresh baby spinach

Directions

1. In a large soup pot, heat the oil over medium heat. Add the onion, cover, and cook until

softened, about 5 minutes. Add the sweet potatoes and broth and cook, uncovered, until the potatoes are tender, about 30 minutes.

2. Ladle about a cup of hot broth into a small bowl. Add the peanut butter and stir until smooth. Stir the peanut butter mixture into the soup along with the cayenne, nutmeg, and salt and pepper to taste.

3. About 10 minutes before ready to serve, stir in the spinach, and serve.

Parsley-Lime Pasta

Preparation Time: 20 minutes

Serving: 4

Ingredients:

- 2 tbsp butter
- 1 lb tempeh, chopped
- 4 garlic cloves, minced
- 1 pinch red chili flakes
- ¼ cup white wine
- 1 lime, zested and juiced
- 3 medium zucchinis, spiralized
- Salt and black pepper to taste
- 2 tbsp chopped parsley
- 1 cup grated parmesan cheese for topping

Directions:

1. Melt the butter in a large skillet and cook in the tempeh until golden brown.
2. Flip and stir in the garlic and red chili flakes. Cook further for 1 minute; transfer to a plate and set aside.

3. Pour the wine and lime juice into the skillet, and cook until reduced by a quarter. Meanwhile, stir to deglaze the bottom of the pot.
4. Mix in the zucchinis, lime zest, tempeh and parsley. Season with salt and black pepper, and toss everything well. Cook until the zucchinis is slightly tender for 2 minutes.
5. Dish the food onto serving plates and top generously with the parmesan cheese.

Nutrition:

Calories: 326, Total Fat: 24.9g, Saturated Fat:12.9 g, Total Carbs: 6 g, Dietary Fiber:1g, Sugar: 4g, Protein: 20g, Sodium: 568mg

Coconut Tofu Zucchini Bake

Preparation Time: 40 minutes

Serving: 4

Ingredients:

- 1 tbsp butter
- 1 cup green beans, chopped
- 1 bunch asparagus, trimmed and cut into 1-inch pieces
- 2 tbsp arrowroot starch
- 2 cups coconut milk
- 4 medium zucchinis, spiralized
- 1 cup grated parmesan cheese
- 1 (15 oz) firm tofu, pressed and sliced
- Salt and black pepper to taste

Directions:

1. Preheat the oven to 380 F.
2. Melt the butter in a medium skillet and sauté the green beans and asparagus until softened, about 5 minutes. Set aside.

3. In a medium saucepan, mix the arrowroot starch with the coconut milk. Bring to a boil over medium heat with frequent stirring until thickened, 3 minutes. Stir in half of the parmesan cheese until melted.
4. Mix in the green beans, asparagus, zucchinis and tofu. Season with salt and black pepper.
5. Transfer the mixture to a baking dish and cover the top with the remaining parmesan cheese.
6. Bake in the oven until the cheese melts and golden on top, 20 minutes.
7. Remove the food from the oven and serve warm.

Nutrition:

Calories: 492, Total Fat:26.8 g, Saturated Fat: 12.6g, Total Carbs: 14g, Dietary Fiber:4g, Sugar: 8g, Protein: 50g, Sodium: 1668mg

Tofu and Spinach Lasagna with Red Sauce

Preparation Time: 20minutes

Cooking Time: 45minutes

Serving: 4

Ingredients:

- 2 tbsp butter
- 1 white onion, chopped
- 1 garlic clove, minced
- 2 ½ cups crumbled tofu
- 3 tbsp tomato paste
- ½ tbsp dried oregano
- 1 tsp salt
- ¼ tsp ground black pepper
- ½ cup water
- 1 cup baby spinach

For the low-carb pasta:

- Flax egg: 8 tbsp flax seed powder + 1 ½ cups water
- 1 ½ cup dairy-free cashew cream
- 1 tsp salt
- 5 tbsp psyllium husk powder

For topping:

- 2 cups coconut cream
- 5 oz. shredded mozzarella cheese
- 2 oz. grated tofu cheese
- ½ tsp salt
- ¼ tsp ground black pepper
- ½ cup fresh parsley, finely chopped

Directions:

1. Melt the butter in a medium pot over medium heat. Then, add the white onion and garlic, and sauté until fragrant and soft, about 3 minutes.
2. Stir in the tofu and cook until brown. Mix in the tomato paste, oregano, salt, and black pepper.
3. Pour the water into the pot, stir, and simmer the Ingredients until most of the liquid has evaporated.
4. While cooking the sauce, make the lasagna sheets. Preheat the oven to 300 F and mix the flax seed powder with the water in a medium bowl to make flax egg. Allow sitting to thicken for 5 minutes.

5. Combine the flax egg with the cashew cream and salt. Add the psyllium husk powder a bit at a time while whisking and allow the mixture to sit for a few more minutes.
6. Line a baking sheet with parchment paper and spread the mixture in. Cover with another parchment paper and use a rolling pin to flatten the dough into the sheet.
7. Bake the batter in the oven for 10 to 12 minutes, remove after, take off the parchment papers, and slice the pasta into sheets that fit your baking dish.
8. In a bowl, combine the coconut cream and two-thirds of the mozzarella cheese. Fetch out 2 tablespoons of the mixture and reserve.
9. Mix in the tofu cheese, salt, black pepper, and parsley. Set aside.
10. Grease your baking dish with cooking spray and lay in one-third of the pasta sheet; spread half of the tomato sauce on top, add another one-third set of the pasta sheets, the remaining tomato sauce and the rest of the pasta sheets.

11. Grease your baking dish with cooking spray, layer a single line of pasta in the dish, spread with some tomato sauce, 1/3 of the spinach, and ¼ of the coconut cream mixture.
12. Season with salt and black pepper as desired.
13. Repeat layering the ingredients twice in the same manner making sure to top the final layer with the coconut cream mixture and the reserved cashew cream.
14. Bake in the oven for 30 minutes at 400 F or until the lasagna has a beautiful brown surface.
15. Remove the dish; allow cooling for a few minutes, and slice.
16. Serve the lasagna with a baby green salad.

Nutrition:

Calories: 487, Total Fat:45.3g, Saturated Fat:34.2g, Total Carbs: 13g, Dietary Fiber:3g, Sugar: 2g, Protein: 14g, Sodium:459 mg

Keto Vegan Bacon Carbonara

Preparation Time: 30 minutes + overnight chilling time

Serving size: 4

Ingredients:

For the keto pasta:

- 1 cup shredded mozzarella cheese
- 1 large egg yolk

For the carbonara:

- 4 vegan bacon slices, chopped
- 1¼ cups coconut whipping cream
- ¼ cup mayonnaise
- Salt and black pepper to taste
- 4 egg yolks
- 1 cup grated parmesan cheese + more for garnishing

Directions:

For the pasta:

1. Pour the cheese into a medium safe-microwave bowl and melt in the microwave for 35 minutes

or until melted.

2. Take out the bowl and allow cooling for 1 minute only to warm the cheese but not cool completely. Mix in the egg yolk until well combined.

3. Lay a parchment paper on a flat surface, pour the cheese mixture on top and cover with another parchment paper. Using a rolling pin, flatten the dough into 1/8-inch thickness.

4. Take off the parchment paper and cut the dough into thin spaghetti strands. Place in a bowl and refrigerate overnight.

5. When ready to cook, bring 2 cups of water to a boil in medium saucepan and add the pasta.

6. Cook for 40 seconds to 1 minute and then drain through a colander. Run cold water over the pasta and set aside to cool.

For the carbonara:

7. Add the vegan bacon to a medium skillet and cook over medium heat until crispy, 5 minutes. Set aside.

8. Pour the coconut whipping cream into a large pot and allow simmering for 3 to 5 minutes.

9. Whisk in the mayonnaise and season with the

salt and black pepper. Cook for 1 minute and spoon 2 tablespoons of the mixture into a medium bowl. Allow cooling and mix in the egg yolks.

10. Pour the mixture into the pot and mix quickly until well combined. Stir in the parmesan cheese to melt and fold in the pasta.
11. Spoon the mixture into serving bowls and garnish with more parmesan cheese. Cook for 1 minute to warm the pasta.
12. Serve immediately.

Nutrition:

Calories:456, Total Fat: 38.2g, Saturated Fat:14.7g, Total Carbs:13 g, Dietary Fiber:3g, Sugar: 8g, Protein:16g, Sodium:604 mg

Not-Tuna Salad

Preparation time: 5 minutes

cooking time: 0 minutes

servings: 4

Ingredients

- 1 (15.5-ouncecan chickpeas, drained and rinsed
- 1 (14-ouncecan hearts of palm, drained and chopped
- ½ cup chopped yellow or white onion
- ½ cup diced celery
- ¼ cup vegan mayonnaise, plus more if needed
- ½ teaspoon salt
- ¼ teaspoon freshly ground black pepper

Directions

1. In a medium bowl, use a potato masher or fork to roughly mash the chickpeas until chunky and "shredded."
2. Add the hearts of palm, onion, celery, vegan mayonnaise, salt, and pepper.

3. Combine and add more mayonnaise, if necessary, for a creamy texture. Into each of 4 single-serving containers, place ¾ cup of salad.
4. Seal the lids.

Nutrition:

Calories: 214; Fat: 6g; Protein: 9g; Carbohydrates: 35g; Fiber: 8g; Sugar: 1g; Sodium: 765mg

Red Bean and Corn Salad

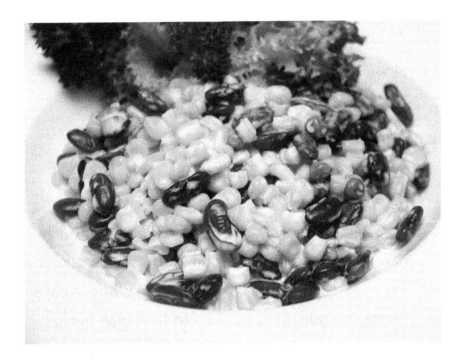

Preparation time: 15 minutes

cooking time: 0 minutes

servings: 4

Ingredients

- ¼ cup Cashew Cream or other salad dressing
- 1 teaspoon chili powder
- 2 (14.5-ouncecans kidney beans, rinsed and

drained

- 2 cups frozen corn, thawed, or 2 cups canned corn, drained
- 1 cup cooked farro, barley, or rice (optional
- 8 cups chopped romaine lettuce

Directions

1. Line up 4 wide-mouth glass quart jars.
2. In a small bowl, whisk the cream and chili powder. Pour 1 tablespoon of cream into each jar. In each jar, add ¾ cup kidney beans, ½ cup corn, ¼ cup cooked farro (if using), and 2 cups romaine, punching it down to fit it into the jar. Close the lids tightly.

Nutrition:

Calories: 303; Fat: 9g; Protein: 14g; Carbohydrates: 45g; Fiber: 15g; Sugar: 6g; Sodium: 654mg

Giardiniera

Preparation time: 15 minutes

cooking time: 0 minutes

servings: 6

Ingredients

- 1 medium carrot, cut into 1/4-inch rounds
- 1 medium red bell pepper, cut into 1/2-inch dice
- 1 cup small cauliflower florets
- 2 celery ribs, finely chopped
- 1/2 cup chopped onion
- 2 tablespoons salt (optional
- 1/4 cup sliced pimiento-stuffed green olives
- 1 garlic clove, minced
- 1/2 teaspoon sugar (optional
- 1/2 teaspoon crushed red pepper
- 1/4 teaspoon freshly ground black pepper
- 3 tablespoons white wine vinegar
- 1/3 cup olive oil

Directions

1. In a large bowl, combine the carrot, bell pepper, cauliflower, celery, and onion.
2. Stir in the salt and add enough cold water to cover.
3. Tightly cover the bowl and refrigerate for 4 to 6 hours.
4. Drain and rinse the vegetables and place them in a large bowl.
5. Add the olives and set aside.
6. In a small bowl, combine the garlic, sugar, crushed red pepper, black pepper, vinegar, and oil, and mix well.
7. Pour the dressing over the vegetables and toss gently to combine.
8. Cover and refrigerate overnight before serving.

Asian Slaw

Preparation Time: 15 Minutes

Cooking Time: 0 Minutes

Servings:4

Ingredients

- 8 ounces napa cabbage, cut crosswise into 1/4-inch strips
- 1 cup grated carrot
- 1 cup grated daikon radish
- 2 green onions, minced
- 2 tablespoons chopped fresh parsley
- 2 tablespoons rice vinegar
- 1 tablespoon grapeseed oil
- 2 teaspoons toasted sesame oil
- 1 tablespoon soy sauce
- 1 teaspoon grated fresh ginger
- 1/2 teaspoon dry mustard
- Salt and freshly ground black pepper
- 2 tablespoons chopped unsalted roasted peanuts, for garnish (optional)

Directions

1. In a large bowl, combine the napa cabbage, carrot, daikon, green onions, and parsley. Set aside.

2. In a small bowl, combine the vinegar, grapeseed oil, sesame oil, soy sauce, ginger, mustard, and salt and pepper to taste. Stir until well blended. Pour the dressing over the vegetables and toss gently to coat. Taste, adjusting seasonings if necessary. Cover and refrigerate to allow flavors to blend, about 2 hours. Sprinkle with peanuts, if using, and serve.

Classic Potato Salad

Preparation Time: 10 Minutes

Cooking Time: 15 Minutes

Servings:4

Ingredients

- 6 potatoes, scrubbed or peeled and chopped
- Pinch salt
- ½ cup Creamy Tahini Dressing or vegan mayo
- 1 teaspoon dried dill (optional)
- 1 teaspoon Dijon mustard (optional)
- 4 celery stalks, chopped
- 2 scallions, white and light green parts only, chopped

Directions

1. Put the potatoes in a large pot, add the salt, and pour in enough water to cover. Bring the water to a boil over high heat. Cook the potatoes for 15 to 20 minutes, until soft. Drain and set aside to cool. (Alternatively, put the potatoes in a large microwave-safe dish with a bit of water.

Cover and heat on high power for 10 minutes.)

2. In a large bowl, whisk together the dressing, dill (if using), and mustard (if using). Toss the celery and scallions with the dressing. Add the cooked, cooled potatoes and toss to combine. Store leftovers in an airtight container in the refrigerator for up to 1 week.

Nutrition Per Serving

Calories: 269; Protein: 6g; Total fat: 5g; Saturated fat: 1g; Carbohydrates: 51g; Fiber: 6g

Brown Rice and Pepper Salad

Preparation Time: 15 Minutes

Cooking Time: 0 Minutes

Servings:4

Ingredients

- 2 cups prepared brown rice
- ½ red onion, diced
- 1 red bell pepper, diced
- 1 orange bell pepper, diced
- 1 carrot, diced
- ¼ cup olive oil
- 2 tablespoons unseasoned rice vinegar
- 1 tablespoon soy sauce
- 1 garlic clove, minced
- 1 tablespoon grated fresh ginger
- ¼ teaspoon sea salt
- ¼ teaspoon freshly ground black pepper

Directions

1. In a large bowl, combine the rice, onion, bell peppers, and carrot.
2. In a small bowl, whisk together the olive oil, rice vinegar, soy sauce, garlic, ginger, salt, and pepper.
3. Toss with the rice mixture and serve immediately.

Avocado Almond Cabbage Salad

Preparation Time: 15 minutes

Cooking Time: 0 minutes

Servings: 3

Ingredients:

- 3 cups savoy cabbage, shredded
- cup ½ blanched almonds
- 1 avocado, chopped
- ¼ tsp pepper
- ¼ tsp sea salt

For Dressings:

- 1 tsp coconut aminos
- ½ tsp Dijon mustard
- 1 tbsp lemon juice
- 3 tbsp olive oil
- Pepper
- Salt

Directions:

1. In a small bowl, mix together all dressing ingredients and set aside.
2. Add all salad ingredients to the large bowl and mix well.
3. Pour dressing over salad and toss well.
4. Serve immediately and enjoy.

Nutrition:

Calories 317 Fat 14.1 g Carbohydrates 39.8 g Sugar 9.3 g Protein 11.6 g Cholesterol 0 mg

Garlic Tahini Spread

Preparation time: 10 minutes

Cooking time: 15 minutes

Servings: 4

Ingredients:

- 1 cup coconut cream
- 2 tablespoons tahini paste
- 4 garlic cloves, minced
- Juice of 1 lime
- ¼ teaspoon turmeric powder
- A pinch of salt and black pepper
- 1 teaspoon sweet paprika
- 1 tablespoon olive oil

Directions:

1. Heat up a pan with the oil over medium heat, add the garlic, turmeric and paprika and cook for 5 minutes. Add the rest of the ingredients, stir, cook over medium heat for 10 minutes more, blend using an immersion blender, divide into bowls and serve.

Nutrition:

calories 170, fat 7.3, fiber 4, carbs 1, protein 5

Baked Hot Spicy Cashews Snack

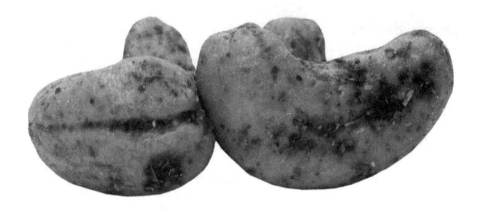

Preparation Time: 20 minutes

Cooking Time: 35 minutes

Servings: 8

Ingredients:

- 2½ c. raw cashews
- 1/3 c. olive oil
- ½ tsp. turmeric powder

- 1 tsp. garlic powder
- 3 c. hot pepper sauce

Directions:

1. In a mixing bowl, mix hot pepper sauce, oil and stir in the turmeric and garlic powder.
2. Add the cashews to the bowl and completely coat with hot pepper sauce mixture.
3. Soak cashews in the hot sauce mixture for several hours.
4. Preheat oven to 325F.
5. Spread the cashews onto a baking sheet and bake for 35-35 minutes.
6. Allow cool and serve.

Nutrition:

Calories: 41, Fat: 29.01g, Carbs: 9.6g, Protein: 6.71g

Spinach and Artichoke Dip

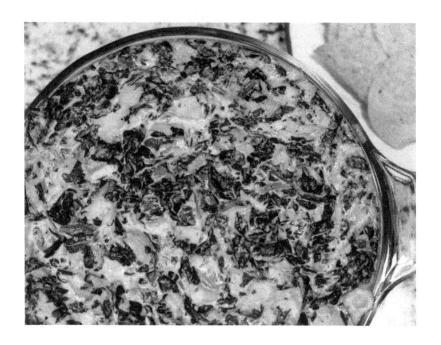

Preparation Time: 10 minutes

Cooking Time: 25 minutes

Servings: 10

Ingredients:

- 28 ounces artichokes
- 1 small white onion, peeled, diced
- 1 1/2 cups cashews, soaked, drained
- 4 cups spinach

- 4 cloves of garlic, peeled
- 1 1 1/2 teaspoons salt
- 1/4 cup nutritional yeast
- 1 tablespoon olive oil
- 2 tablespoons lemon juice
- 1 1/2 cups coconut milk, unsweetened

Directions:

1. Cook onion and garlic in hot oil for 3 minutes until saute and then set aside until required.
2. Place cashews in a food processor; add 1 teaspoon salt, yeast, milk, and lemon juice and pulse until smooth.
3. Add spinach, onion mixture, and artichokes and pulse until the chunky mixture comes together.
4. Tip the dip in a heatproof dish and bake for 20 minutes at 425 degrees f until the top is browned and dip bubbles.
5. Serve straight away with vegetable sticks.

Nutrition:

Calories:124 Cal, Fat: 9 g, Carbs: 8 g, Protein: 5 g, Fiber: 1 g

Cocoa Muffins

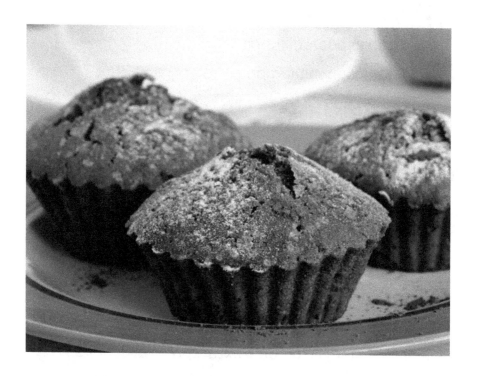

Preparation time: 10 minutes

Cooking time: 25 minutes

Servings: 6

Ingredients:

- ½ cup coconut oil, melted
- 3 tablespoons stevia
- 1 cup almond flour

- ¼ cup cocoa powder
- 3 tablespoons flaxseed mixed with 4 tablespoons water
- ¼ teaspoon vanilla extract
- 1 teaspoon baking powder
- Cooking spray

Directions:

1. In bowl, combine the coconut oil with the stevia, the flour and the other ingredients except the cooking spray and whisk well.
2. Grease a muffin pan with the cooking spray, divide the muffin mix in each mould, bake at 370 degrees F for 25 minutes, cool down and serve.

Nutrition:

calories 344, fat 35.1, fiber 3.4, carbs 8.3, protein 4.5

Coconut Salad

Preparation time: 10 minutes

Cooking time: 0 minutes

Servings: 6

Ingredients:

- 2 cups coconut flesh, unsweetened and shredded
- ½ cup walnuts, chopped
- 1 cup blackberries
- 1 tablespoon stevia
- 1 tablespoon coconut oil, melted

Directions:

1. In a bowl, combine the coconut with the walnuts and the other ingredients, toss and serve.

Nutrition:

calories 250, fat 23.8, fiber 5.8, carbs 8.9, protein 4.5

Pear Mincemeat.

Preparation Time: 35 Minutes

Servings: 6

Ingredients:

- 4 firm ripe Bosc pears, peeled, cored, and chopped
- 1 large orange
- 1½ cups apple juice
- 1¼ cups granola of your choice
- 1 cup raisins (dark, golden, or a combination
- 1 cup chopped dried apples, pears, or apricots, or a combination
- ½ cup packed dark brown sugar or granulated natural sugar
- ¼ cup brandy or 1 teaspoon brandy extract
- 2 tablespoons pure maple syrup or agave nectar
- 2 tablespoons cider vinegar
- ½ teaspoon ground cinnamon
- ½ teaspoon ground allspice
- ½ teaspoon ground nutmeg
- ¼ teaspoon ground cloves

- Pinch of salt

Directions:

1. Zest the orange, then peel it, deseed it, and quarter it.
2. Blend the orange flesh and zest and put in your Cooker.
3. Add the pears, dried fruits, juice, sugar, brandy spices, vinegar, and salt.
4. Seal and cook on Stew for 12 minutes.
5. Release the pressure naturally, take out some of the juice, then reseal and cook another 12 minutes.
6. In a bowl mix the granola and syrup.
7. Release the pressure of the Cooker naturally and sprinkle the crumble on top.
8. Seal the Cooker and cook on Stew for another 5 minutes.
9. Release the pressure naturally and serve.

Mango Rice Pudding.

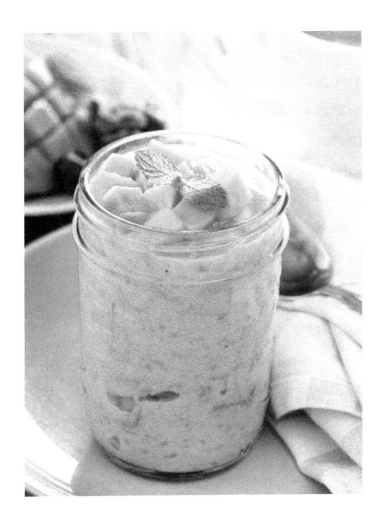

Preparation Time: 35 Minutes

Servings: 6

Ingredients:

- 2 (14-ouncecans unsweetened coconut milk
- 2 cups unsweetened almond milk, plus more if needed
- 1 cup uncooked jasmine rice
- ½ cup granulated natural sugar, or more to taste
- 1 large ripe mango, peeled, pitted, and chopped
- 1 teaspoon coconut extract
- 1 teaspoon pure vanilla extract
- ¼ teaspoon salt

Directions:

1. Spray the Cooker insert with cooking spray.
2. Add the milks and bring to a boil.
3. Add the rice, sugar, and salt, seal, and cook on Rice.
4. Depressurize quickly and stir in the extracts and mango.
5. The pudding will thicken as it cools.

Poached Pears In Ginger Sauce.

Preparation Time: 25 Minutes

Servings: 6

Ingredients:

- 2½ cups white grape juice
- 6 firm ripe cooking pears, peeled, halved, and cored
- ¼ cup natural sugar, plus more if needed
- 6 strips lemon zest
- ½ cinnamon stick
- 2 teaspoons grated fresh ginger
- Juice of 1 lemon
- Pinch of salt

Directions:

1. Warm the grape juice, ginger, lemon zest, salt, and sugar until blended.
2. Add the cinnamon stick and the pears.
3. Seal and cook on Stew for 12 minutes.
4. Take the pears out.
5. Add lemon juice and more sugar to the liquid.
6. Cook with the lid off a few minutes to thicken.
7. Serve.

Maple & Rum Apples.

Preparation Time: 25 Minutes

Servings: 6

Ingredients:

- 6 Granny Smith apples, washed
- ½ cup pure maple syrup
- ½ cup apple juice
- ⅓ cup packed light brown sugar
- ¼ cup golden raisins
- ¼ cup dark rum or spiced rum
- ¼ cup old-fashioned rolled oats
- ¼ cup macadamia nut pieces
- 1 teaspoon ground cinnamon
- ½ teaspoon ground nutmeg
- Juice of 1 lemon

Directions:

1. Core the apples most of the way down, leaving a little base so the stuffing stays put.
2. Stand your apples upright in your Cooker. Do not pile them on top of each other! You may

need to do two batches.

3. In a bowl combine the oats, sugar, raisins, nuts, and half the nutmeg, half the cinnamon.

4. Stuff each apple with the mix.

5. In another bowl combine the remaining nutmeg and cinnamon, the maple syrup, and the rum.

6. Pour the glaze over the apples.

7. Seal and cook on Stew for 20 minutes.

8. Depressurize naturally.

Mint Rice Pudding

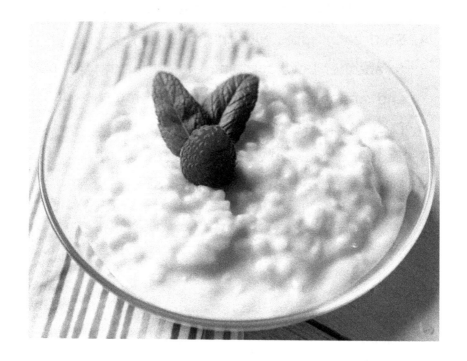

Preparation time: 10 minutes

Cooking time: 30 minutes

Servings: 4

Ingredients:

- ¼ cup stevia
- 2 cups cauliflower rice
- 2 cups coconut milk

- 2 tablespoons walnuts, chopped
- 1 tablespoon mint, chopped
- 1 teaspoon lime zest, grated
- ½ cup coconut cream

Directions:

1. In a pan, combine the cauliflower rice with the stevia, the coconut milk and the other ingredients, whisk, bring to a simmer and cook over medium-low heat for 30 minutes.
2. Divide the pudding into bowls and serve.

Nutrition:

calories 200, fat 6.3, fiber 2, carbs 6.5, protein 8

Almond Fat Bombs

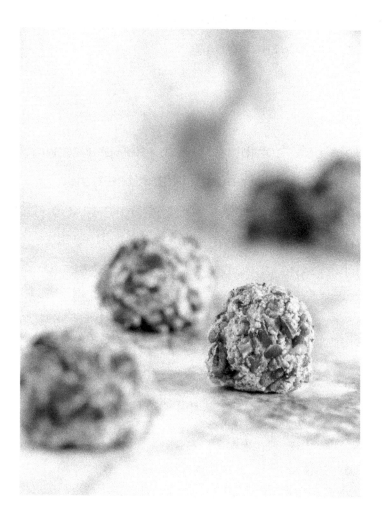

Preparation Time: 10 minutes

Cooking time: 25 minutes

Servings: 7

Ingredients:

- 1 cup almond flour
- 2 tablespoon Erythritol
- 1 teaspoon vanilla extract
- ¼ cup coconut butter
- 1 tablespoon almonds, crushed

Directions:

1. In the mixing bowl combine together almond flour and crushed almonds.
2. Add Erythritol, vanilla extract, and coconut butter.
3. Use the fork and knead the smooth and soft dough. Add more coconut butter if desired.
4. After this, make the medium size balls with the help of the fingertips and place them in the fridge for at least 25 minutes.
5. When the fat bombs are solid – they are cooked. Store the dessert in the fridge up to 5 days.

Nutrition:

Calories 156, fat 13.2, fiber 3.3, carbs 10, protein 4.2

NOTE

CPSIA information can be obtained
at www.ICGtesting.com
Printed in the USA
BVHW091345100621
609271BV00003B/609